The AIDS Awareness Library™

What Is AIDS?

Anna Forbes, MSS

The Rosen Publishing Group's
PowerKids Press™
New York

To Arran, 9, and Carl, 7, and all of their generation.
May they live to see the cure.

Published in 1996 by The Rosen Publishing Group, Inc.
29 East 21st Street, New York, NY 10010

First Edition

Book design: Erin McKenna

Photo credits: Cover © Michael P. Manheim/International Stock; p. 4 © L. J. Schnieder/International Stock; p. 7 © E. Sander/Gamma Liaison; p. 8 by Yung Hee Chia; p. 11 © Peter Russell Clemens/International Stock; p. 12 © P. Perrin–Figaro Magazine/Gamma Liaison; p.15 by Maria Moreno; p. 16 © Stefan Lawrence/International Stock; p. 19 © Hal Kern/International Stock; p. 20 © Richard Shock/Gamma Liaison.

Forbes, Anna, MSS
    What is AIDS? / Anna Forbes.
        p.   cm. — (The AIDS awareness library)
    Includes index.
    Summary: Presents information about the disease called AIDS by explaining such things as what causes it, how it is spread, and how to avoid getting it.
    ISBN 0-8239-2368-1
    1. AIDS (Disease)—Juvenile literature. [1. AIDS (Disease). 2. Diseases.] I. Title.
RC607.A26F6326 1996
616.97'92—dc20
                                                       96-5879
                                                          CIP
                                                           AC

Manufactured in the United States of America

Contents

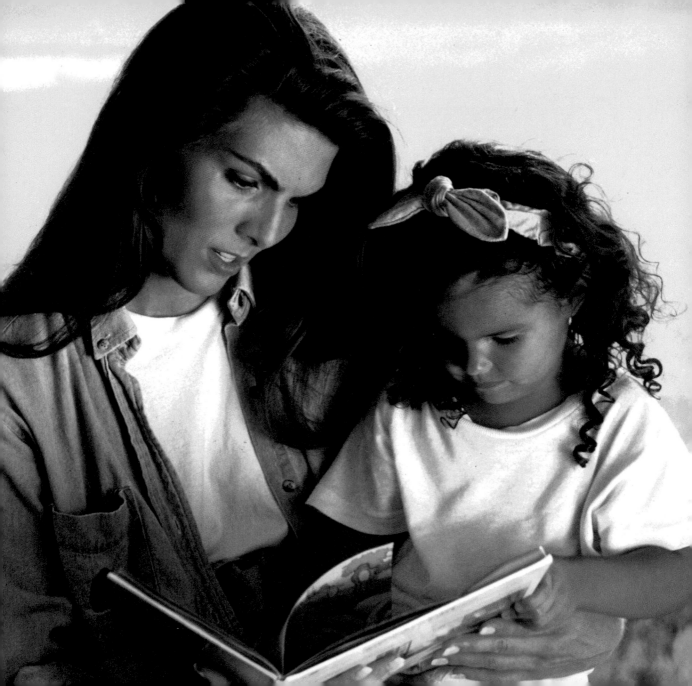

A Disease Called AIDS

This is a book about a **disease** (diz-EEZ) called AIDS. By the end of 1995, half a million people in the United States had AIDS. About 300,000 people have died from it. You may know someone who has it. Or you may know someone who died from it.

Thinking about AIDS may be scary or sad. But knowing the facts may help you feel less scared. Knowing the facts about AIDS can help you keep yourself safe.

◀ Knowing the facts about AIDS can help you feel less scared of it.

What Is AIDS?

AIDS has only been around for about 20 years. It wasn't even called AIDS until 1981. Before then, doctors knew that a new disease was making people sick. They also knew that people could die from it. But they didn't know what the disease was. Some doctors thought it was one kind of disease. Others believed it was another kind. AIDS wasn't quite like anything else. In 1981, AIDS was given its own name because doctors finally agreed that it was a completely new disease.

In 1981, doctors finally agreed that ▶
AIDS was a new disease.

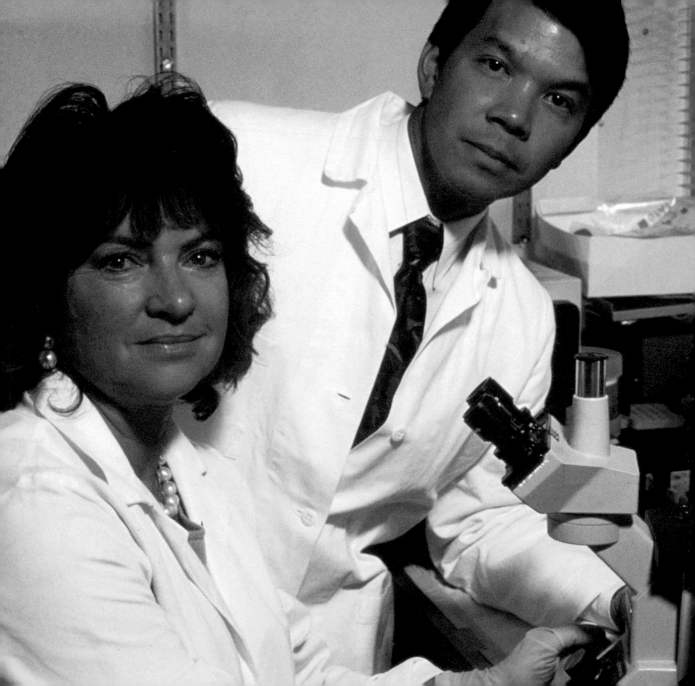

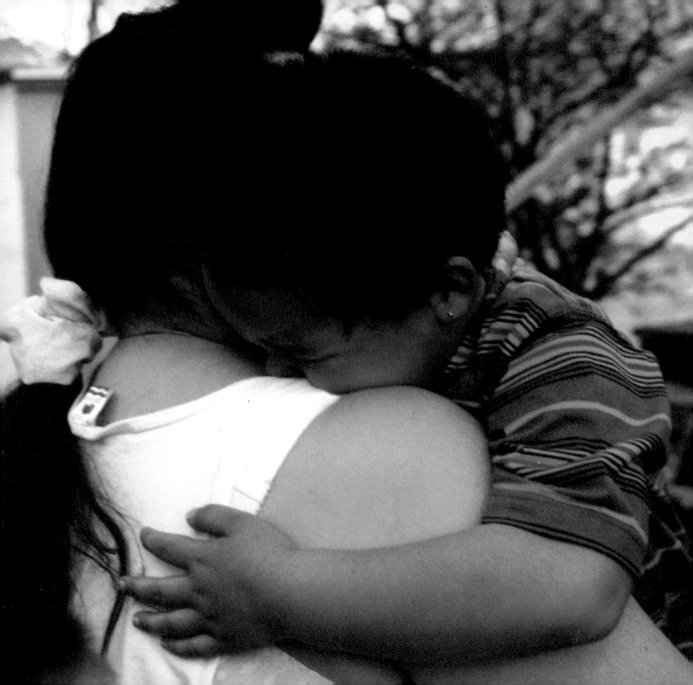

What Does AIDS Mean?

AIDS stands for **acquired** (uh-KWYRD) **immunodeficiency** (im-MYOO-no-dee-FISH-en-see) **syndrome** (SIN-drome). Acquired means something that you get, like a cold. Most people with AIDS got it by having sex in an unsafe way or by sharing unclean needles, especially when using drugs. Some people have gotten AIDS from someone who has HIV or AIDS by getting that person's blood in their blood by accident. Other people with AIDS were born to a mother who had HIV or AIDS.

◀ Some kids were born to a mother who had HIV or AIDS.

Immunodeficiency

Immunodeficiency means that AIDS makes the **immune system** (im-MYOON SIS-tem) in our bodies weak.

Blood is made up of tiny parts called cells. Each type of cell has a job to do. Immune system cells keep us healthy by fighting off germs or **viruses** (VY-rus-sez). Most of the time our immune system cells win, and we don't get sick. But the AIDS virus kills immune system cells. So people with AIDS have weak or **deficient** (dee-FISH-int) immune systems.

People with weak immune systems get sick a lot. ▶

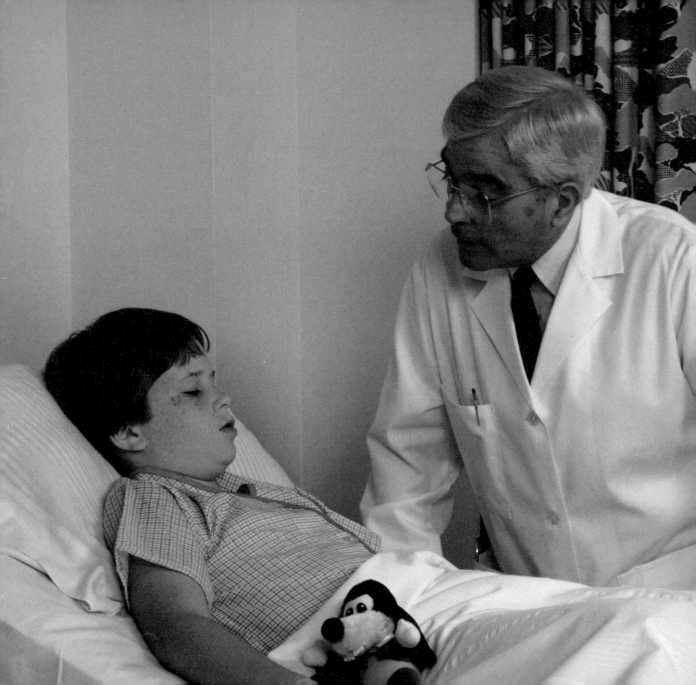

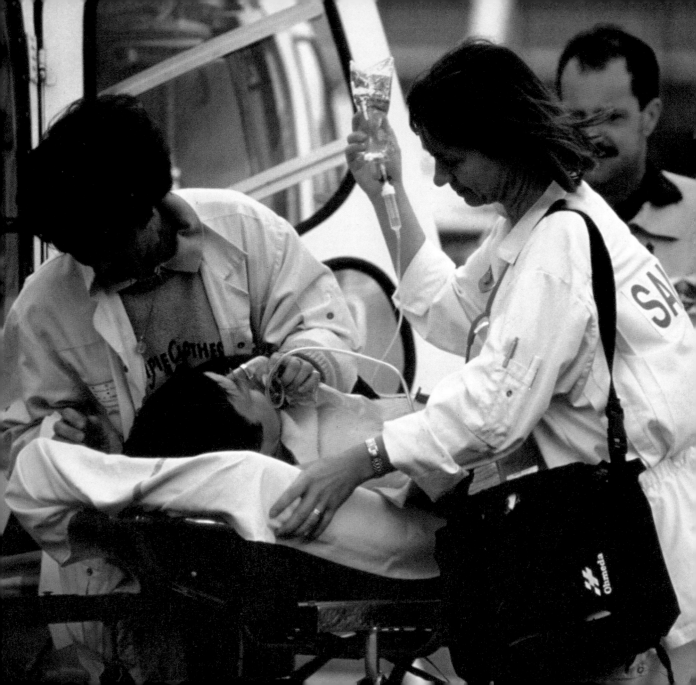

What Is a Syndrome?

The last letter in AIDS stands for syndrome. A syndrome means several illnesses that all happen together.

AIDS isn't just one sickness like measles or mumps. People with AIDS have weak immune systems. This means that they can get sick a lot. Some of the illnesses are mild, such as colds or sore throats. But some of them are very serious, such as **pneumonia** (new-MOAN-ya) or **cancer** (KAN-ser).

◀ Some illnesses people get when they have AIDS are very serious.

What Causes AIDS?

A virus called HIV can cause AIDS. HIV stands for human immunodeficiency virus.

Human means that only humans get it. Animals don't get HIV. Immunodeficiency means having a weak immune system. And a virus is a type of germ that causes disease.

You can't tell just by looking at someone if he or she has HIV. ▶

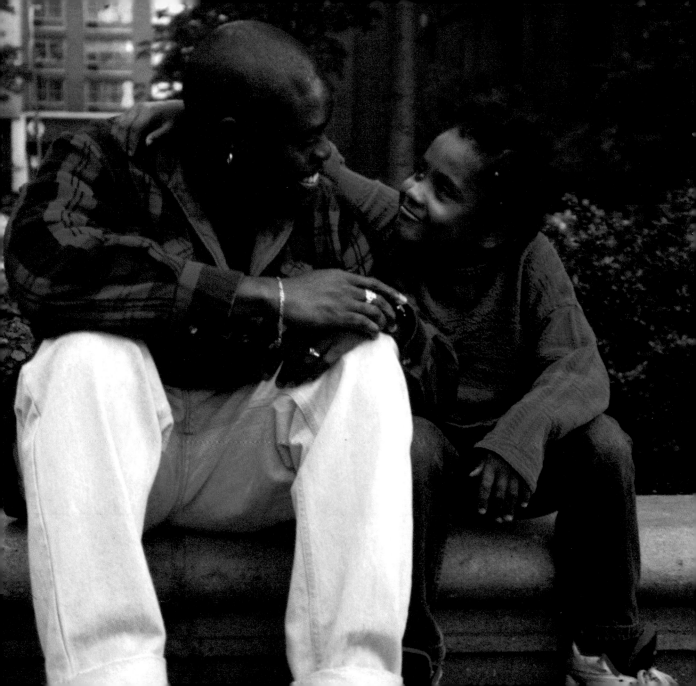

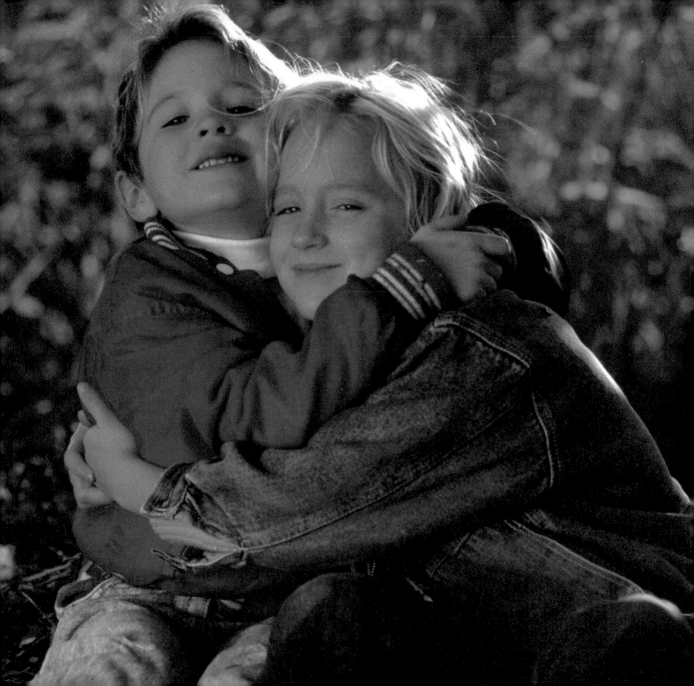

Where Does HIV Live?

HIV lives only in human blood and in the body fluids that grown-ups produce for having sex. It can travel from one person to another only when two people have sex or if one person's blood mixes with the blood in another person.

HIV doesn't live in saliva, tears, sweat, or **urine** (YUR-in). You can't get HIV if someone with HIV or AIDS coughs or sneezes on you. And you can't get it from hugging or kissing a person with HIV or AIDS.

◀ You can't get HIV or AIDS by hugging or playing with someone.

Do Kids Get AIDS?

Most people get AIDS from having unsafe sex or by sharing needles to use drugs. Since most kids don't have sex or use drugs, most kids don't get HIV or AIDS. Almost everyone with AIDS is grown-up.

Most kids who do have HIV or AIDS were born with it. Before birth, all babies share their mother's blood supply. If a mother has HIV or AIDS, her blood can carry HIV to her baby. Her baby may then develop AIDS.

Most children who have AIDS were born with it. ▶

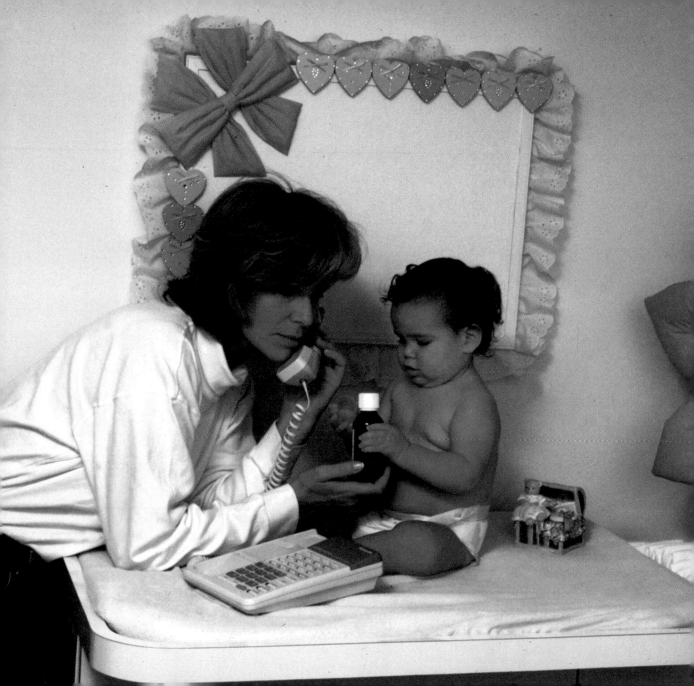

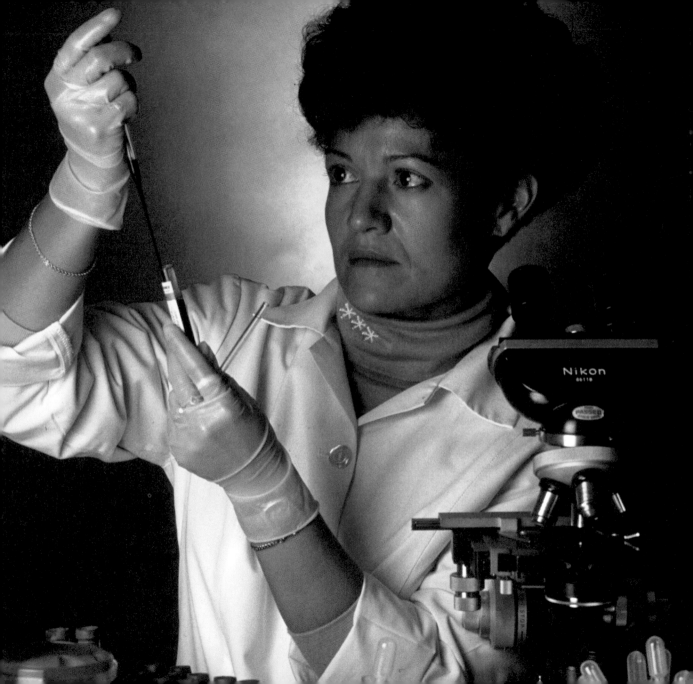

Is There a Cure for AIDS?

Right now there is no cure for AIDS. Doctors and scientists are looking for drugs to stop HIV and cure AIDS. They've found some drugs that seem to help people with HIV and AIDS to get sick less often. But they haven't found a cure yet.

◀ Scientists are working hard to find a cure for AIDS.

What Can We Do?

There are three things that we can all do about AIDS.

- Don't use drugs or have unsafe sex.
- Tell other people what we know about the disease.
- Help people who have HIV or AIDS by being friendly and kind.

By doing these three things, you can help other people understand HIV and AIDS and how to stay safe.

Glossary

acquired (uh-KWYRD) Having gotten something.

cancer (KAN-ser) Serious disease that can sometimes cause death.

deficient (dee-FISH-int) Not strong; weak.

disease (diz-EEZ) Illness caused by a virus or germ.

immune system (im-MYOON SIS-tem) How our bodies fight off disease.

immunodeficiency (im-MYOO-no-dee-FISH-en-see) Having a weak immune system.

pneumonia (new-MOAN-ya) Serious disease affecting the lungs that can sometimes cause death.

syndrome (SIN-drome) Several illnesses happening at the same time or one right after the other.

urine (YUR-in) Bodily waste; pee.

virus (VY-rus) Germ that causes disease.

Index